WEIGHT LOSS AND WELLNESS

By: Susanna Karlen

SUSANNA KARLEN

The information herein is offered for informational purposes solely and is universal as so. The presentation of the information is without a contract or any type of guarantee assurance.

The trademarks that are used are without any consent, and the publication of the trademark is without permission or backing by the trademark owner. All trademarks and brands within this book are for clarifying purposes only and are owned by the owners themselves, not affiliated with this document.

DISCLAIMER

The Author and Publisher have strived to be as accurate and complete as possible in the creation of this book, although he does not warrant or represent at any time that the contents within are accurate due to the rapidly changing nature of the Internet. While all attempts have been made to verify information provided in this publication, the Author and Publisher assume no responsibility for errors, omissions, or contrary interpretation of the subject matter herein. Any perceived slights of specific persons, peoples, or organizations are unintentional. In practical advice books, like anything else in life, there are no guarantees of results. Readers are cautioned to rely on their own judgment about their individual circumstances and act accordingly. This book is not intended for use as a source of legal, medical, business, accounting, or financial advice. All readers are advised to seek services of competent professionals in the legal, medical, business, accounting, and finance fields.

Table Of Contents

CHAPTER 1: AN INTRODUCTION TO WEIGHT LOSS

Weight loss is a critical problem of today's general population with growing obesity, and people increasingly understanding what being overweight is doing to their health, their well-being, and their lives.

For other circumstances, weight loss is beneficial. It is of genuine benefit in diabetes, hypertension, shortness of breath, joint problems, and elevated cholesterol.

Weight loss is conceivable through healthy diets of your own, but having high-quality protein and bulk incline construction can make you lose much further, allowing you to hold your weight off and remain strong.

Weight loss is guaranteed on an out-of-chance basis that one adheres to the regulation of the eating routine.

Weight loss essentials: consume more calories than you need, add on weight; use more than you use, and lose it. Weight reduction is a goal that will become fully successful if we stick to the planning policy, to abstain from diet arrangements. Be that as it may, surgery can be the only concern for a few.

Surgical techniques have progressed in recent decades, and most of them are convincing because they typically result in a fast and substantial decrease in weight.

In any case, all specialists agree that the ideal approach to maintaining weight loss is to take after a healthy lifestyle. Whatever approach you take, the path to long-haul achievement is a moderate, consistent weight loss. It is shown that it is essential to prepare yourself mentally for your journey of weight loss and that the way of life changes you are going to experience.

For morbidly obese patients, surgery to side-step portions

of the stomach and small digestive tract will now again be the most effective strategy for producing a sustainable once substantial weight loss.

A long-lasting responsibility for general exercise and sensible dietary patterns is a key factor in achieving and maintaining weight loss. You will find that your life levels are enhanced by weight loss, which brings you so much individual fulfillment.

Drinking water is one of the best weight loss tips that dieticians give to people and produces an extra 100 + calories a day. Per twenty soda pops that you lose from your usual admission is like a weight loss of around one pound.

Fasting: While fasting has a significant effect on a few eating practices, it is generally not recommended for healthy weight loss. Fasting can lead to low blood sugars, headaches, weakened immune systems, and even more serious problems.

Diet

Dietitians are nutritionists who consult directly with clients or patients to fulfill their health needs. Abstaining from food decreases the caloric intake; however, exercising requires you to consume more calories. Eat fewer carbs. It's better than you ever imagined to eat fewer calories. With a veggie-lover to eat fewer calories, weight loss shouldn't be a matter of concern.

It is recommended that decreased calories will refrain from food containing moderate fat. Consideration of different organic foods for weight loss feeding methodologies is a good method for managing hunger. Additionally, giving the body the supplements and vitamins that it needs legitimately to function.

Workout while you diet: Weight loss is all about reducing your caloric intake while going to increase the calories that you want to burn. Above all, choose how much weight you need to lose and set yourself, preferably with the aid of your dietitian or expert, a reasonable goal.

A diet that works for a couple of people might not work for others. Quick breakfast is one of the main elements of a balanced diet and a dramatic decrease in weight. Most eating patterns, if taken completely, will cause weight loss due to calorie control.

Much of the early weight loss on eating food with low calories, burns weight from muscle tissue and not fat.

Upwards of 85 percent of calorie counters that don't exercise all the time recover their pounds shed within two years. Over- and above weight loss and regeneration (yo-yo calorie counting) encourages the body to store fat and raise the chance of a patient contracting cardiovascular disease.

Eating three balanced dinners a day-with a simple supper in the early afternoon is a more effective solution to forecasting corpulence than fasting or collapsing diets, which convinces the body that hunger is on the rise.

Individual lifestyles, sustenance inclinations, longings, all should be considered when building a dietary arrangement. The sustenance instructor needs to tailor the person's eating routine, rather than receive a "one-measuring fits-all" approach. Lesser fat eating methodologies can be the strongest within a week of weight loss. Being overweight is a result of an insufficient measure of work out, a lack of lifestyle routine, and an inadequately balanced eating schedule for a significant number of people.

Many high-fiber foods are similarly rich in water and low in calories, allowing them to eat less starch. Dissolvable fiber will decrease cholesterol; it contains insoluble fibers that add bulk to our weight management strategies.

Drinking water is one of the best weight loss tips that dieticians give to people and produces an extra 100 + calories a day.

A decisive guide to eventual achievement: regular workout and a balanced diet. Add one day of sticking to your diet schedule to save yourself from cravings.

Eat a healthy diet packed with bunches of vegetables, organic products, and whole-grain items.

Fasting: Although fasting has a significant influence on a few dietary regimens, it is mostly not prescribed for safe weight reduction.

Surgery

In any case, for some in this situation, surgery for weight loss is the greatest choice. Gastric sidestep surgery was one of the earliest devices. Nowadays, there are many types of surgery, all of which have upsides and downsides.

Nevertheless, there are still accommodating risks, as with any big operation. To people who consider surgery to be the only option, advice from a doctor is vital.

Today, most surgeons prefer to perform laparoscopic surgery because it is negligibly obtrusive.

You're able to add form and muscle to weight quotients in the unlikely risk that you're going to lose your pounds and eat calories in the middle of normal daily practices. It has a cellular effect on the body, which allows fat cells to discharge their fat away to be copied as vitality. The food you consume in the middle of the day will be scorched away by activity.

Exercise when you diet: Weight tragedy is about reducing your caloric consumption when you maximize the calories you burn. Eating less decreases your food consumption, but exercising lets you eat more calories.

As a result, we know that to maintain a healthy weight reduction, we need to eat a greater amount of calories than we do. Exercise increases the metabolic rate by creating a muscle that consumes more calories than fat.

At a time when general exercise is consolidated with predictable, stimulating dinners, calories continue to burn at a faster rate for a few hours. Calories burned, relying on your level of activity.

Not only do fats give you a feeling of completion, but eating enough sound fat called omega-3 unsaturated fats can make your digestion system even more productive. On the off chance that your weight will remain steady, you are most likely to take the same amount of calories you burn every day.

If you slowly lose weight for some time, your caloric entry is greater than the number of calories you burn from your day by day workouts.

The amount of calories that we burn every day depends on our basic metabolic rate (BMR), the number of calories that we burn every hour, essentially by being alive, and keeping our body's capacity and our level of physical movement.

Our weight also assumes a part in deciding what number of calories we are still burning, more calories are needed to keep your body in its present express, the more prominent your body weight. Someone whose job involves overwhelming physical work will burn a higher number of calories per day than someone who sits in the work area for the vast majority of the day (inactive occupation).

The number of calories consumed can be increased in people who do not have jobs requiring extraordinary physical action, training, or increased physical movement.

To lose one pound, you're supposed to burn about 3500 calories far beyond what you're doing as you burn every day. Use a calorie add-on machine to make sense of how many calories you burn while sitting, standing, working, lifting weights, and so on. If you're eating fewer calories than you're burning, you're going to lose your pounds.

Because it's outstanding when the body doesn't get enough calories, the fat stored in the fat tissue begins to burn.

Exercise will help you burn overabundance of calories and fat, tone and make muscles as well.

CHAPTER 2:I'M DOING EVERYTHING RIGHT, BUT I'M STILL NOT LOSING WEIGHT. WHAT'S GOING ON?

Rewind three-and-a-half months to January. You've woken up, feeling the after effects of last night's celebration, and resolved to make a change in the new year. The goal? To lose weight. Fast forward to today. You've cut out the fast food, revamped your diet and committed to an exercise routine. But the numbers on the scale haven't budged at all. What gives?

You're following a weight-loss eating plan. You're exercising almost every day. You're proud of the new healthy habits you've learned. Yet week after week, the scale barely seems to budge. What gives?

Chances are your food portion sizes have crept up (time to get out the scales and measuring cups again). Or your workouts may not be quite as intense as you think (start checking that heart rate).

But if you know you've followed your reducing plan religiously, there's another possibility: A medical condition -- or medication -- may be to blame.

If you haven't been able to lose weight and you can't understand why, you need to determine whether there's a medical condition underlying your weight problem, You need to cure that problem first before you can address the weight issue.

Medical Reasons for Weight Gain

Several conditions can cause weight gain or hinder weight loss, says Rebecca Kurth, MD, director of PrimeCare at Columbia-Presbyterian Eastside and associate professor of clinical medicine at Columbia University.

Among them, Kurth says, are:

Chronic stress : When you live with anxiety, stress, or grief, your body can produce chemical substances -- like the hormone cortisol -- that make your body more likely to store fat, especially around the waist. That's the type of weight gain that really increases your risk of serious health problems. (Extra weight around the hips and thighs poses fewer health risks.)

Cushing's syndrome : This happens when the adrenal glands (located on top of each kidney) produce too much cortisol, which leads to a buildup of fat in the face, upper back, and abdomen.

Hypothyroidism : If your thyroid is underactive, your body may not produce enough thyroid hormone to help burn stored fat. As a result, your metabolism is slower and you will store more fat than you burn -- especially if you're not physically active.

Polycystic ovary syndrome (PCOS): This disease, the result of a hormonal imbalance, afflicts more than 5 million women in the US. Common symptoms are irregular menstrual bleeding, acne, excessive facial hair, thinning hair, difficulty getting pregnant, and weight gain that is not caused by excessive eating.

Syndrome X: Also called insulin resistance or hyperinsulinemia (high insulin levels), syndrome X goes hand-in-hand with weight gain. Syndrome X is a cluster of health conditions thought to be rooted in insulin resistance. When your body is resistant to the hormone insulin, other hormones that help control your metabolism don't work as well.

Depression : Many people who are depressed turn to eating to ease their emotional distress.

Hormonal changes in women: Some women may gain weight at times in their lives when there is a shift in their hormones -- at puberty, during pregnancy, and at menopause.

Two other considerations: people tend to gain weight with age for unknown reasons, and though it's not a medical condition, drinking alcohol in moderate to excessive amounts can sabotage your efforts to lose weight. Alcohol (including beer and wine) is a refined carbohydrate, similar to sugar, candy, and white flour. Besides adding calories, alcohol may raise blood sugar and insulin levels, which can contribute to weight gain.

Fat Burning Foods For Women and Men

There's no doubt that burning fat is the answer to weight loss and a healthy look. Many diet and fitness experts argue that there are plenty of fat-burning foods for women and men that move the whole process much faster forward. If you can learn to recognize and eat those foods in the way you should, you can tell giant steps forward on your fitness journey, and you will be eating many of the foods that you love.

Believe it or not, some of the foods you thought you could never have on any diet are often encouraged on diets that promote fat burning weight loss. Like any fad, diets change from day to day, and while it was once thought that eating the fat of any kind was a bad thing, research has shown that we have to eat fat to stay healthy and lose weight. The secret lies in knowing which fats to eat and which ones to avoid. Many men and women have lost weight following plans that target mainly belly fat, as it is one of the most stubborn areas.

Here is a brief description of the five best fat burning foods for women and men alike who want to lose belly fat specifically as well as achieve successful overall weight loss.

Olives

Olives are a great source of healthy unsaturated fats that also provide lots of iron, Vitamin E and copper, and contain healthy doses of fibre that aid in blood sugar control and a healthy digestive tract.

Oils

Olive oil especially contains many properties that promote good health, and when used regularly, in the right amounts can improve weight loss efforts. Other beneficial oils include safflower, canola, walnut, and sunflower oil.

Nuts and seeds

Seeds of sunflower, almonds, walnuts, and even pistachio nuts will help you burn fat and lose weight when eating as scheduled. Nuts also provide a good protein source and lots of different vitamins and minerals.

Avocados

A lot of people who love this buttery treat avoid it when trying to lose weight or burn fat when they should be eating even more of it! Like the other monounsaturated fats listed here, avocados promote fat loss when incorporated into a planned fat loss diet. So the next time you toss that super salad, be sure to add a few avocado chunks for good measure!

Dark Chocolate

Now here is the best news yet for those seeking fat burning foods for women and men! Dark chocolate is good for you and can help you lose weight and burn fat!! So you'll have to give up some of those television snacks, but if you can eat chocolate, things are not going to be that bad. Once again, while it's a healthy fat, it also needs to be consumed in moderation.

In conclusion, the secret to burning fat and losing weight is about exercise, eating the right foods, in the right amounts, and the right combination. It isn't rocket science; it's mostly just about using common sense, moderation, perseverance, and following a plan that works for you and your lifestyle.

Women Baby Boomer and The Four Keys to Weight Loss

As a Baby Boomer woman, I realize that the pressures of career, family, and daily life over the years all too often mean that our health and well-being, our time to care for ourselves, can get lost in the shuffle. When thinking, "I'm not going to have time for that right now" or "I 'm going to get around to that later," it's too simple to put off doing stuff for oneself. Whether you've had trouble losing the extra weight and keeping it off with dieting or if you've just got a weight on it, the dilemma is the same. How do we make the decision and the commitment to be healthier and, finally, succeed with our health goals?

The metabolism was probably higher when we were younger than it is now. We weren't putting on weight as fast, and we could lose weight with less effort. Once we were younger, we could get away with sketchy eating habits; but if you're like most people in Baby Boomer, you 're dragging overweight around. Those extra pounds can mean a future of deteriorating physical ability, diabetes, cancer, or heart disease. This is no way you should spend the rest of your life. Looking back on your life, I 'm confident you've achieved some goals. What if you could be creating a future where your # 1 goal is good health? What does it take to get you there? Here are four keys to your aim:

1. Figure what you wish for. How do you feel like living the rest of your life? Get Clear and Specific. Wanna be more physically fit? Need to have as much flexibility and freedom as possible? What weight would you like to lose? What if you'd want to have what? I think you can.

2. Make a list of everything that you get from getting to

your goal. This will motivate you along your journey, and entice you. What will allow you to do, have and be that important to you to lose the weight and be more fit?

3. Make the decision that you want to have and commit to doing what it takes. Decide to do it now, not later. In the end, you 're responsible for your weight and your health. It's time for a break. Don't put off your good health anymore. Imagine your future, if you do not prioritize your wellbeing.

4. Enable. Health and weight loss are along many routes. Whether with a weight loss clinic, online support, a mentor for weight loss, or with friends, find out what works best for you. Decide what small steps you will constantly take with your safe goal in mind along the way.

Make yourself a Baby Boomerang Boomerang! You keep coming back to your target with sustained effort until you achieve your balanced, ideal body. Be consistent, diligent, and committed. They 're going to be worth it. You can have the gift of looking back over your life, knowing you've done what it took. You made time for yourself, achieved better health, and became a role model to follow for others. Go on-Baby Boomer Girls-teach us how this happens!

Walking, Water, and Weight Watchers:

I've been working seriously on weight loss for about 2 1/2 months, and many people have asked me what I'm doing to make it so successful. I reply, "The 3 W's for weight loss!" Of course, they don't know what the 3 W's of weight loss are, so I promptly tell them, "Walking, Water, and Weight Watchers." I know that's not a formula that's going to work for everyone, but it works for me! Water is an essential fluid that everyone needs, walking is an excellent form of exercise, and Weight Watchers is a world-renowned weight-loss organization, which has helped millions of people lose weight and keep it off for good.

Walking:

Walking is a feel-good calorie-burning exercise that most of us have been doing for the majority of our lives. Besides a good pair of running boots and comfortable clothing, no other equipment is needed, so the price is right! Perhaps the most amazing thing about walking is the advantages it provides for your wellbeing. Strolling is easy on joints, and in certain people, it relieves back pain. It is capable of lowering blood pressure, lowering cholesterol levels, reducing the risk of diabetes and heart disease, building muscle and strengthening bones, and leading to weight loss! Try to walk 10,000 steps or more every day!

So far, I've lost 24 1/2 pounds, but aside from the weight loss, walking every day allows me to relax mentally, and I feel it lowers my stress levels. The funny thing is, the more I walk, the more my mind and body seem to be craving it. For me walking is a very healthy habit.

Water-Water:

New research showed this after a 17 oz cocktail. All men and women reported a 30 percent rise in their metabolic rate of water, which lasted about 40 minutes.

A few months ago, I stopped soda and replaced it with water. I can already sense a difference in my skin tone, and that helps with my weight loss efforts, of course as it fills me up, and I am less likely to eat too much. Drinking water every day is a habit now and because of that, I feel much better! Beverage 8, 8 oz. Water glasses to improve your weight loss efforts every day!

Weight Watchers:

Weight Watchers was created by Jean Nidetch in the early 1960s. She started by holding small informal meetings in her home to address weight loss issues. Those small meetings have expanded over the years and now, Weight Watchers has evolved into a global movement made up of millions of people committed to the weight loss mission.

Weight Watchers is a science-based program that encourages weight loss through positive lifestyle changes to improve mental, emotional, and physical wellbeing. Weight Watchers meetings are structured to provide weight-loss inspiration, diet and exercise statistics, and a relaxed atmosphere in which participants and leaders provide shared support and encouragement. There are hundreds of meeting places around the world, and Weight Watchers are now also available online.

My Weight Watchers leader is awesome, and I look forward to my meeting every week. And that she's a wonderful role model, having shed 45 pounds on herself, but she also has the innate capacity to bring out the best of all of us who are regularly attending her meetings. She surrounds herself with medical research, her own weight loss story, motivational quotes, fitness tips, and recipes; she wraps in a warm sense of humor to give us the resources we need for the coming week.

When you were disappointed with previous efforts to lose weight, try the 3 W's of weight loss. It is a good way to lose weight, and I'm sure the results will please you!

CHAPTER 3:QUICK WEIGHT LOSS WITH EXERCISE

In order to achieve quick weight loss with exercise you will have to do a lot in a short time. You will have to, naturally, adopt a very rigorous regimen of working out, and possibly dieting. This ain't no easy to take weight loss pill or any other form of easy weight loss. Instead it is predicated on both discipline and hard work: not exactly things that we like to just pick up and run with like that. Nevertheless, I am here to give it to anyone straight who wants to achieve such "overnight" results. It certainly is possible. It's not even that hard really. Most of the blockage is in one's own mind, and nowhere else. I suppose this is the case with any method of safe weight loss, including these forms of hyper exercise that I am about to describe.

The first in our series of exercises to lose weight is rigorous aerobic routines. These don't have to last more than an hour or so, but they do have to put a major healthy strain on your body. This is the basis of any real program which hopes to achieve quick weight loss with exercise for you. Aerobics moves through the whole body, and really starts to get it toned in a very natural way. It pulls, stretches, and tones the muscles. It can be, too, a fun way to lose weight. The human body naturally rejoices at such a hearty movement. I'm sure you have had this experience in the past and can draw upon it in order to bring your current goals into fruition.

Let's face it: weight control is not easy under most circumstances. But if you take this hard-working but quick approach to it, you can use its limited period and quicker results in order to motivate you.

Other exercises I would suggest are sit-ups, push-ups, pull-ups (if you can do them), possibly some form of weight lifting in order to give your body more capability in whatever methods you choose to try to burn those calories. Just by doing these things on a daily basis, and pushing yourself, you should see that quick weight loss with exercise is indeed an achievable goal.

Fast weight loss with exercise is possible, depending on your weight loss goals. Let's look at how you can do it and shed those pounds.

The body burns fat from a difference between energy put into the body through eating and energy that the body needs to supply fuel to the muscles and bodily functions.

If the energy it needs to operate is more than the energy in the food we eat, then the body kicks into fat burning mode to make up the difference.

Hence, exercise is about the only way to put more demand on the body for energy consumption above and beyond your normal daily routine.

The best weight loss with exercise is achieved when you put your body into its "fat burn" zone of operation and keep it there for a while without interruption.

The fat burn zone of your body will depend on your gender and your age. Check with your local gym. They usually have charts that show you the heart rate range for your age group.

The best fat burn zone for your body will be between 60% and 75% of your maximum heart rate as indicated by the chart.

Here is something to remember. When you exercise at the rate where your heartbeat is in that range, you should still be able to carry on with normal speech. You should not be so out of breath that you have trouble talking or have to gasp for air. If you have to do that, slow down, you're overdoing it.

It is important to keep your body in that zone of operation for at least 30 minutes. Your body only begins to burn fat after a good 10 to 12 minutes of exercise. During that time, it first consumes the immediate nutrition that is available to it.

For fast weight loss with exercise you will probably need to go for longer than 30 minutes. An hour to ninety minutes would consume a sizeable chunk of fat every day.

Once again, do not overdo it. Doing this for three hours a day is probably going to be worse than better. One disadvantage is it is going to leave you completely exhausted.

Also accelerate your metabolism while you are exercising like this. You do that by eating six to seven small meals per day.

Remember, whenever you're exercising and you start feeling

dizzy, nauseous, or experience pain or discomfort, stop immediately and consult with your physician.

Fast weight loss with exercise is not worth pushing yourself beyond your physical limits and causing your body to suffer serious damage.

Eating and weight loss go hand in hand

While you're on the weight loss route, forget all about the false promises you'll hear on the midnight infomercials or the new 'miracle pill' bottle. There is no instant miracle solution when it comes to losing weight. To lose weight effectively and healthily, you need to eat a balanced diet as well as exercise. People have lost weight by starving themselves, true, but this is not healthy and will only bring harm to your body. You will also have to understand how your body uses food and how calories are burned and stored.

Your Body Is A Finely Tuned Machine

How our body works is truly amazing. The food that we eat is nothing more than the fuel used by the body to give us energy, to repair itself, and to protect us. This is where the fat comes in. Your body does not know that society deems fat as ugly and un-attractive. Your body stores excess calories as fat to protect you from the cold, as insulation and cushioning to your muscles, bones, and internal organs. Your body also stores fat if you ever face starvation, since it stores as energy just in the case you are faced with a dire situation. Once you understand all that, you can see how you can use the way your body uses food to your advantage. Nutrition and weight loss is all about balance and eating the right amounts of food, at the right time, to prevent the excess calories from being stored as fat.

If You're Already Overweight

If you're reading this and you're overweight, you'll need to balance your diet to weight loss. That means you should eat plenty of fruits and vegetables, plenty of protein, and diet nutritional supplements like a fat burner to make the process faster and give you more power. And you've got to add some workout to your routine of course. If you want to push your metabolism into high gear, you need to get a sufficient amount of exercise. If you consume smaller meals more often, your appetite will be continually activated, and your fat will burn faster if you add exercise to the mix. Burning will increase until you find yourself losing weight before you know it.

Nutrition and weight loss are easy to maintain. You just have to keep a schedule, at least only at first. You wouldn't have to feel like you're on a diet, being too rigid to sound like the plan you 're on. You just need to make a change in life. Keeping a schedule might include eating every two or three hours, always working out in the morning first thing in the morning before breakfast, or it could be something as simple as working out on Mondays, Wednesdays, and Fridays. By keeping your schedule, you are more likely to stick with it, which is essential to weight loss through nutrition.

Gradual Change

The thing with weight loss is that it happens gradually. Results don't appear overnight, so it is going to take some time. Make a schedule, keep a routine, and try to forget that you are on a diet, and you're in a nutrition and weight loss plan; just make it a part of your lifestyle. One day you will notice that you feel better, your clothes feel.

Pregnancy Diets and Weight Loss

The single factor that lets down mothers is their excess weight after pregnancy. First of all, weight gain at the time of pregnancy cannot be controlled, and it has to be reduced later, which is toilsome. Pregnancy diets and weight loss becomes imperative during motherhood. Gaining weight for the period of pregnancy is quite a stable process. So, the reduction of fat should be in the same way without giving any sort of stress or strain to the body.

Many women are unaware of the fact that breastfeeding can assist in weight loss. It is the natural way of the body to get rid of the unwanted fat. At this instant, when it comes to pregnancy diets and weight loss, visit your gynecologist and hunt for advice in support of accurate knowledge of weight loss.

Pregnancy diets and weight loss ought to be accompanied by workouts. It will rally round you to drop those additional pounds produced for the duration of pregnancy, lighten postpartum gloominess and, dissimilar to dieting, and it won't get in the way with your breastfeeding. Women who do not feel pretty easy with workouts can ultimately move on to pregnancy diets and weight loss.

A hale and hearty diet is the most excellent technique to misplace your pregnancy pounds.

Have a discussion with the general practitioner concerning what provisions are significant for your infant's long-lasting physical condition. Concentrate on nourishment, not on plain fad diets. Another major thing is that weight loss comes automatically after delivery. Just take care without gaining too much weight.

The majority of medical doctors give an opinion to by no means challenge weight loss, at the same time as pregnant. It is vital to accommodate an adequate amount of calories and nutrients, as the baby requires plenty of energy and power to survive. Pregnancy diets and weight loss that harshly controls calories or put a ceiling on precise food collections are putting you out of bed for an unfit baby and perhaps pregnancy difficulties.

Another major misconception is that pregnancy means weight gain to many, which is quite wrong. Eating healthily rather than too much of fatty food is normal enough for the mother as well as the baby. It does denote that pregnancy diets and weight loss demand to be looked at cautiously to ensure appropriate nutrition for both.

If there is one part on a woman's body that most of us normally don't like, it is the upper arms. They can look soft and 'mushy,' or flabby, or even have fat that causes those unkind names -- bingo wings, or bat wings, or lunch-lady arms.

Arms we can't be proud of is more common as women get older, but it's also common among women of any age who have lost a lot of weight. Having upper arms that aren't toned will prevent you from wearing short sleeve shirts, tank tops, or strapless dresses. There's also the issue of wanting to have more arms (and upper body) strength. The good news is that with the

Shake Weight for Women and in just six minutes per day, you can start to get those arms toned again, and it doesn't take long to see results.

How Does the Shake Weight for Women Work?

This is a special product because it is lightweight and does not demand that you go and lift huge dumbbells or barbells. It's easy enough to do it yourself at home, which means you won't need a pricey membership in the gym to get the workout you need or the time to get to the gym to make the expensive membership worthwhile.
The Shake Weight for Women works by using "dynamic inertia," which is just a term to describe the rapid action and how it works your muscles, helping to increase your muscle activity by nearly 300 percent over what you would get with dumbbells of the same weight. These statistics are scientifically proven, and as soon as you try this out, you will be able to see just how intense this workout can be.

Is It Easy to Do? Does it hurt?

Learning the motion that you need to do is easy, but working out is not. You will need to devote a full six minutes (eventually) to using the weight, but because this also comes with an included DVD that shows the correct form and three exercises, that time will pass quickly. Either way, it is still a lot easier than a half-hour in an aerobics class, for more benefit!
Users say they thought it looked easy, but it isn't. You will feel it - but that's how you know it's working!

What Will Shake Weight for Women Do for You?

If you are tired of having flabby arms, this is the only product on the market that is completely designed to get them toned up and also add shoulder, back, and core strength (including your abs). While it can't remove hanging skin (often caused by very rapidly losing a lot of weight; this may require surgery to correct), it can strengthen and tonearms for most women. The fact that you can use the Shake Weight for Women while you are watching television or even during a work break at the office is an added benefit.

CHAPTER 4:WEIGHT LOSS DIETARY SUPPLEMENTS - WHAT WORKS QUICKLY?

Weight loss dietary supplements promise a quick way to loose weight. But more than just quick, they also promise an easy way to loose weight. As we search for a way to appease our desire for instant gratification, we often slip right by the one thing that would work and show results quickly.

The primary appeal for weight loss supplements is in the quick and easy solution they offer to those of us trying to loose weight. This appeal is difficult to ignore because it catapults us to our end goal faster than we can probably get there without it.

There is a great emotional tug behind a product that promises to work fast whether you get off the coach or not, whether you stop driving to fast food stores or not, that is often is too great for many of us to ignore.

The problem is that in taking a short cut to loose weight, we are not acknowledging the patterns in our life that caused us to gain weight in the first place.

For example, I had an unhealthy pattern of eating quick and easy to prepared foods that were over processed and filled with carbohydrates and sodium. Yes, weight loss dietary supplements might have helped me loose weight, but they would not have lowered my cholesterol (raised by the high levels of sodium).

The best way to get fast results in your weight loss efforts is to develop a mindset that accepts results when it sees them.

Are you waiting until you loose 30 lbs before you congratulate yourself? Are you sure that your efforts are worthless unless you have dropped three clothing sizes?

Consider that when you begin to eat fewer processed foods and include more natural foods in your diet, you are experiencing instant success. When you get off the couch and begin to walk around your local area a few times a week you are experiencing yet more success.

Big demands like losing all the excess weight or looking like you did as a teenager seem so far off in the future that dietary supplements almost seem like a necessity.

Divine Link Between Faith and Weight

Do the words trust and weight go together to achieve success? They do, I guess. Faith will inspire your efforts to achieve achievement through weight and give you spiritual energy to keep working when you want to give up. There are many things we could do to raise our weight-loss goals. We have to remain emotionally linked, even though it affects our weight. You have supernatural power, so why not use it?

Tapping into divine power will mean the difference between success and failure. When it comes to leading a healthier and happier life, you should blend divine energies with your eating plan, fitness activities, and attitude. I figured that was important to me.

There have been times in my life that I have faced certain issues, and the first thing I wanted to do was satisfy my feelings. But I was focusing on leading a healthier and happier lifestyle, and I knew it was no longer an option to fuel my emotions. I was going to seek God for his help to deal with things that I was doing, and I realized that inner strength was flowing out.

I had to learn how to supplement my unhealthy eating habits with better eating habits, and religion played a large part in that. Even Religion helped me crack from emotional eating. It took a long time to know that perhaps I could not eat away my suffering. There were times when I would pray and give me a sense of peace and security that it wasn't consuming. I've also learned things like how to unleash positive thinking about weight loss, how to believe more in myself, self-love, meditation strategies, and other important pieces to the weight success puzzle.

When it comes to thinking about my religion, I'm not nervous, so when people I meet ask me how I lost the weight, I still share that religion plays an important role. Although I had not, I wouldn't sound real. Faith made me see where I was and where I needed to go beyond. Faith has helped me unleash the hope I needed to remain focused. Faith let me know that not being perfect was Okay. Faith let me know that I can still get back on track even when I made eating mistakes. And faith let me know I could succeed by weight. For me, there is a connection between faith and weight success, for which I will always be grateful.

Surprising Link Between a Good Night's Sleep and Weight Loss

Whether you're trying to lose weight, you've probably made changes to your diet and start exercising also. But there's another lifestyle change that you need to make and one you might not expect. A new study finds there appears to be a connection between sleep and weight loss - those who slept less than 6 hours a night (short sleepers) tended to be heavier than those who got more sleep.

Though the work was small, involving only 14 nurses, it analyzed the sleep, activity, and energy levels of the volunteer subjects who were part of a heart health initiative known as the Integrative Cardiac Health Project.

The patients provided diet therapy, fitness preparation, stress control, and sleep recovery as part of the curriculum. The nurses often wear special bracelets that assessed how busy they were, their location in the body, and other measures of action and rest.

When evaluating the data by grouping the subjects into

'short sleepers' and 'long sleepers,' the findings revealed that short sleepers appeared to have a higher BMI, 28.3 kg/m2, relative to long sleepers had an average BMI of 24.5.

There was also poorer sleep output for short sleepers, observed as greater trouble getting to sleep and staying asleep.

A normal BMI measurement falls between 18.5-24.9, while BMI of 25.0-29.9 is considered overweight, a BMI of 30.0 or over falls into the obese category. You can find out where you stand by using one of the many handy online BMI calculators.

What's interesting is that overweight participants were more active than the normal subjects in the study, taking an average of 13,896 steps a day vs. 11,292 for the normal-weight women. That's almost a 25% difference. The overweight subjects also burned 1,000 more calories a day (3,064 vs. 2,080) than the normal weight subjects.

The trouble is all that extra energy expenditure didn't show itself on the scale, which left the team wondering if sleep might somehow have a part to play in weight loss.

For now, no one is sure why sleep might impact weight, but there are some interesting theories.

Lack of sleep might throw off natural hormone balance (leptin, the satiety hormone, for example) that would trigger overeating.

Lack of sleep also is known to make our bodies more ready and willing to store fat. And since your body works best when it is well-rested and fully recharged, lack of restorative sleep can keep you from having the energy for workouts.

What's more, too little sleep makes handling everyday stress, stuff like flat tires and lost lunches, that much more of a challenge. Little things make you crazy, and your fuse is shorter, so you're more likely to reach for comforting, calorie-laden foods as a way to cope.

Experts also know that stress can start a chain of biochemical processes - storing fuel, slowing down metabolism, and releasing chemicals like cortisol, leptin, and other hormones linked to obesity. All reasons why the research team is planning to continue to work to try and uncover the potential connection between sleep and weight loss.

The role of body shape in losing weight and regaining weight

When you go on a diet for weight loss, something strange happens. Your body isn't able to lose its fat entirely. You continue losing lean tissue, including muscle and bone mass, then.

A research study in Denmark reported in May 2002 in the American Journal of Clinical Nutrition found that when men died, less than 60 percent of the weight lost was fat. The remainder were lean tissues. Just 24 percent of the weight they put back on after men regained weight was lean tissue-more than 75 percent of the weight recovered following weight loss was more fat. That means people who eat yo-yo-live in a loop of weight loss and adding it back on again-are slowly replacing the lean tissues in their bodies with fat.

The same study has found that the scenario is much worse for women! During the diet, lean tissue was 35 percent of the weight lost-initially less than for men. Yet on regaining weight, lean tissue was just 15 percent. When women lost weight and then regained, lean tissue was not properly preserved-85 percent of the regained weight was obese!

Looking a little deeper at the issues of how body composition is key to preventing weight regain, the facts are clear - the vast majority of people who deliberately lose weight put it back on again! Regardless of how much weight is lost, research shows that a full 95% of all weight is put on again within five years. The same research links weight regain to body composition. So what's going on?

The crux of this problem lies in the different ways in

which lean tissue cells and fat cells function in the body.

Every cell in your body has a specific function - nerve cells, brain cells, heart cells, skin cells, even fat cells all have a particular job to do, and they are programmed to do it! Now we don't need to understand all those functions - we just need to understand two things. Lean tissue cells burn energy - they use the calories in the food we eat. Fat cells store energy - they burn none of the calories that we consume. So the fewer lean mass cells we have, the fewer calories our bodies burn before they are stored as body fat.

Let's do a simple bit of maths! Imagine a body that needs 2000 calories a day, just to function. Taking out any lean tissue by food, and the body requires less than 2000 calories a day to work at the end of the meal, as it has fewer cells than can consume fat. To follow the same routine of eating as before the diet means that the body actually cannot use as many calories as before the diet for weight loss and retain the surplus as fat. Yeah, the presto-the body takes on more pounds effortlessly and quite instantly as soon as a weight loss program comes to an end, and daily meal service is restored!

Being aware of this makes all the difference - both during and after the weight loss program itself.

By choosing a weight loss program that preserves your lean tissues, you can make sure your body composition doesn't suffer. By maintaining lean tissues throughout weight loss, you ensure you keep the cells with the ability to burn the calories in the food you eat. So when you have reached your target weight, your body still needs the same number of calories afterward as it did before the weight loss program.

Have you ever followed a diet where it seems harder and slower to lose weight as you progress? That's possibly an indicator that you are losing significant amounts of lean tissue. As you follow your program, your body can tolerate fewer and fewer calories before weight loss starts to grind to a halt, to stop, and even to reverse! Your body can only shed actual fat slowly - the faster the weight loss, the faster you lose lean tissues instead of fat! To stop this loop of weight loss and rebound, you have to resist unrealistic strategies that guarantee you huge and fast weight loss - don't maintain restraint during the weight loss phase, and you'll pay the latter in-lbs of fat for rehabilitation!

Once you reach your target weight, you still need to be mindful of the types of food you eat, even though you can have more of it! By knowing which nutrients slow down the rate at which calories are released into the body, you can make sure that the energy from those calories can be used steadily by the lean tissue cells to fuel their various functions before it is stored as fat again.

There are multiple factors involved in healthy weight loss and healthy weight regain. In summary, the number of calories is not the only factor to be considered: what those calories are made of is crucial to preserving, or even promoting health through weight loss.

CHAPTER 5:HOW TO SUPPLEMENT: TIPS FOR HEALTHY WEIGHT LOSS AND APPETITE CONTROL

When it comes to healthy weight management, it's all about striking the right balance between exercising and eating a nutritious diet. If you want to lose weight in a healthy way and need help keeping your appetite in check, an easy to use daily system with lean protein and supplements to fuel your weight loss can provide support to help you reach your goals.

FIGHT CRAVINGS AND CUT CALORIES

Keep your calorie count down and fight temptations by incorporating meal replacement shakes and bars into your diet program. The protein in them provides you with energy and will help keep you feeling fuller longer. Plus, they're a convenient, nutritionally balanced way to control your portions and your calories. To manage your calorie intake and keep yourself feeling full, look for bars, powders and shakes with approximately 25 grams of protein, three grams of fiber and no more than 200 calories. You can use them to supplement smaller meals throughout the day or replace one or two of your meals.

TONE AND SCULPT

Daily diet aids can jumpstart your weight loss goals. Taking a CLA supplement can help support a healthy body composition. CLA is conjugated linoleic acid, a naturally occurring fatty acid that can help you fuel energy and fat metabolism and improve lean muscle tone. When taken daily and used in conjunction with regular exercise and a healthy diet, CLA can enhance your diet and support your metabolism. Thermogenics, both ca eine-driven and non-stimulant, have the potential to help increase metabolism and fuel fat-burning workouts.

COUNTER NUTRITIONAL GAPS

When you're cutting calories and certain foods from your diet, you can inadvertently cut out important vitamins and nutrients in the process. Taking a multivitamin daily with food can help fill nutritional gaps as you diet. Carnitine—found in red meat – fuels fat metabolism and can be supplemented to support weight loss goals, especially in diets focused on vegetarian protein sources. While more than one daily pill or capsule can seem like a lot to remember, Vitapak® Programs conveniently deliver pre-packaged, customized nutrition for your goals in an easier way to consistently use every day.

Even if working on water balance is a part of your weight management plan, don't forget to pay extra attention to your hydration when starting any new fitness routine or diet. Supplying your body with the nutrients and water it needs to feel energized and strong is an important component of every healthy weight loss program.

Feel Better, Look Great

A growing number of health and medical authorities support the notion that there is a link between black cohosh and weight loss, especially among women during PMS. According to various sources, regular intake of black cohosh aids weight loss efforts indirectly because it stabilizes hormonal fluctuations that can spur women to overeat.

These hormonal fluctuations usually occur during PMS and menopause. They lead to a host of symptoms such as menstrual pain, hot flashes, and other difficulties that women have to struggle with. Under these conditions, a lot of women resort to eating for temporary relief or to replenish lost energy, which has been spent trying to cope with hormonal difficulties. These are the make or break days of women in their daily battle against weight. During days when they struggle the most, many women decide to junk their diets and calorie counts for a day or two to quickly regret their decision. Black cohosh aids weight loss efforts because it alleviates many of the symptoms of hormonal fluctuations and, therefore, lessens the inclination to eat.

Black Cohash's Healing Properties

Black cohosh is a natural herb that has been regarded as a powerful natural medicine for centuries. At that time, it has been ascribed to have health and healing properties. It derives its name from its appearance - black because its root is colored black and 'cohash' because that means 'rough.' The root is widely believed to be the source of this herb's potency. Nutritionists and health professionals believe the black cohosh root contains many powerful nutrients and chemicals that rival the effectiveness of the most modern pharmaceuticals today. There is now growing evidence that links black cohosh and weight loss.

During premenstrual syndrome, black cohosh is believed to alleviate menstrual difficulties such as pain, hot flashes, muscle spasms, cramps, and other symptoms of hormonal change because it bolsters the flow of blood and makes women better equipped to handle PMA. Besides, black cohosh helps women relax and focus on their weight loss program without distractions.

Women are less prone to lose track of their diet or cheat a little, telling themselves that they need that extra energy or that positive boost that food can bring to help them cope with PMS. When you're suffering, you tend to embrace anything that can take your mind off the pain, even for a little while. Eating is a logical choice. But thanks to black cohosh, your weight loss program does not have to be sacrificed for a little relief.

Increased Blood Flow Burns Fat

Health professionals also believe the relationship between black cohosh and weight loss may stem from the herb's capacity to increase blood flow to the muscles, which, in turn, can increase oxygen in these muscles. Fat burns when it is exposed to oxygen. Therefore by indirectly increasing oxygen in the muscles, black cohosh helps burn fat.

Birth Control Pills and Weight Control

The Oral Contraceptive Pill (OCP)

A subset of birth control compounds called hormonal contraception refers to the Oral Contraceptive Pill (OCP) or birth control pill. The underlying science behind them is the disruption of the natural release of the female hormones that contribute to ovulation, or development of an egg. If no egg is released, fertilization can not occur. OCPs can also facilitate milder, more regular periods, and some control conditions, such as endometriosis. In the United States, the overwhelming majority of females use OCPs at some point in their lives. A large-scale study of women in America recently reveals that about 82 percent of women in this age range have used OCPs at any stage between the ages of 15 and 44, and at any given time, about 20 percent of women in this age range use OCPs. Due to side effects such as headaches, mood changes, and weight gain, between 20 and 60 percent of women will stop using OCPs. Many hormonal contraceptives list the changes in weight as a side effect. This point of this piece is on discussing OCPs and gaining weight.

Weight gain-what the study says: There is a good body of evidence showing that most women will undergo little or no weight gain from OCPs relative to women who do not use hormonal regulation or any other process. The section explains many such studies:

- A study using teenagers measured weight gain in OCP patients instead of getting depot medroxyprogesterone acetate (Depo-Provera). It found no significant weight gain for OCP users, but those using the depot injection nevertheless saw some significant weight change. Later on, weight gain and deposit are discussed.

- No weight gain was due to OCPs or NuvaRing for three months in the O'Connell analysis described above.

- In a test intended to determine why women stopped using OCPs, the majority of OCP consumers did not gain weight. About 20 percent of the study participants gained weight, but more than 75 percent either lost weight or did not undergo any improvement.

-- Another adolescent study grouped the users by weight starting. Participants were then divided into groups using Depo, OCPs, or no hormonal contraceptives but grouped into either non-obesity or obese categories. In this study, the use of OCP was associated with no weight gain in the category obese and a smaller increase in the category of healthy weight than non-hormone users. The non-obese and obese girls who do not use hormones gained more weight (7 to 8 pounds in a year and a half) than any group of users of OCP. Obese OCP users gained less than half a pound, while non-obese OCP users gained 6 lbs.

The bottom line is that there is no evidence from a significant number of recent reports that obese or non-obese women are receiving weight gain by using an OCP.

What's up with Depo?

Deposit Medroxyprogesterone acetate represents a particular form of hormonal contraception. An injection is given to users every three months, and no pills are taken. Several studies have shown users a significant increase in body weight, which appears to be worse for heavier women in sharp contrast to OCPs. An earlier study in 1995 compared women who had used three forms of pregnancy hormones and noted marginal body weight differences. Thus, there may be a select number of girls with a time putting on weight easier than the depot's average user. This category may represent people who get heavier as the use of the depot starts.

The bulk gained less than 5 percent of their original weight in a study comparing OCP customers with Depot. A significantly larger number of Depot users gained > 10 percent of their starting weight. People taking birth control pills appear to experience little or no weight gain due to the drug, and those using Depot may be at higher risk of gaining weight.

 But note-by increasing your activity level (daily steps, short walks, exercise, etc.) and eating fewer calories, you can always avoid weight gain or lose weight.

CHAPTER 6:HOW TO OVERCOME COMMON WORKOUT FEARS AND FINALLY LOSE WEIGHT

Easy solutions for feeling self-conscious in the gym, battling back pain and other common workout concerns that prevent you from losing weight.

Are workout fears keeping you from the gym? Getting back into an exercise routine is daunting enough, let alone joining a new facility that you are unfamiliar with, surrounded by people you don't know.

A nationwide survey of 1,000 Americans conducted by Fitrated found that 65 percent of women and 36 percent of men avoid the gym out of fear of being judged. This apprehension was more common among those who rated themselves less attractive, less in shape or less experienced at the gym than others. And the fears may not be completely unfounded: one in three respondents admitted to judging others while at the gym.

In addition to feeling self conscious about how you look or your fitness level, uncomfortable physical sensations and fear of injury can all add additional layers of anxiety that can make it hard to motivate ourselves to get to the gym.

But if you're making fitness a priority in the new year, we're here to help you bust through some common fears that may be holding you back — and ease that mental burden a bit.

Fear: Feeling Self-Conscious About How You Look

Over half of people surveyed by Fitrated admitted to not looking fit enough to be at the gym, and nearly 44 percent said they felt judged for their clothing choice. But you don't need to go out and drop a chunk of change on a new workout wardrobe to feel better. If you're wearing an oversized t-shirt, you can tuck it in in the front or roll up the sleeves to give it some shape. If you're not happy with what your body looks like right now, you can also use a few tricks to hide trouble spots you might be uncomfortable with. If you're embarrassed by flabby arms, wear a long-sleeve dry-fit workout shirt over a sports bra (instead of a short-sleeve shirt with a jacket over it, which is too likely many layers for an indoor workout).

Professional stylist Samantha Brown recommends looking for garments with a thick, stretch fabric or even compression fabrics to help slim the body. "Quality matters here, as higher end athletic lines are designed with more attention to hiding loose skin, cellulite and silhouettes that flatter," she says. When it comes to downplaying certain areas of your body, she recommends to "look for matte fabrics (avoid shine and glossy materials). While pattern will draw the eye, a darker print can also help to minimize the appearance of cellulite or loose skin tone as it provides distraction." She also says, "to help downplay a loose tummy, opt for a high-waisted legging or athletic pant with a wide band. Anything low cut exaggerates this problem area."

After a few minutes on a cardio machine, you may feel out of breath, and maybe you panic. I had a client who explained this fear to me multiple times — saying that she knew it was inevitable to get out of breath, but she couldn't push past it. She felt silly, but she'd simply get off the machine when the breathing got difficult because she was so scared of not being able to breathe altogether.

Dr. Jamie Wells, director of Medicine for the American Council on Science and Health, explains that it's not uncommon to get out of breath with exercise, especially if you're out of shape. She encourages people to have "a fully informed conversation with and possible evaluation by your doctor, because going instantly from extremes of a more sedentary lifestyle to a heavy duty workout tends to cause the most problems. Easing into it is likely more enduring and will be a more ideal bet."

So remember not to go from zero to 100 right out of the gate. As you're working out, check in with your breathing. Breathe in through your nose, and blow out through your mouth. Do some self-talk and tell yourself that you will be okay if breathing starts to become more challenging (and that you can always get off the machine). Start by giving yourself a 1-minute time period to be out of breath. If it's too difficult to bust through this fear on your own, hire a personal trainer for one session with the goal of getting out of breath while supervised.

And it is smart to be aware of signs that may be worrisome. "Those concerning signs include, but are not limited to, chest heaviness or pressure especially with a rapid heart rate, inability to catch your breath, lightheadedness or feeling faint, chest pain, confusion, feeling like your heart is racing as well as dizziness along with poor color," says Dr. Wells.

Fear: Breaking a Sweat

I once had a client who was so scared of breaking a sweat that we had to put a wet washcloth on her neck during her workouts. She felt comfortable sweating if it was hot outside, but not comfortable making herself sweat at the gym. With the washcloth, I was able to help her focus her attention on being cool on a sensitive spot on her body (her neck) while the rest of her body was sweating. Sweating is one of your body's ways of detoxing, so we also continued to focus on the positive effects of sweating (instead of the discomfort).

Wells explains, "We sweat as a normal way to self-regulate our body temperature and dissipate heat should we be taxed by physical exertion or hot weather, for example. An otherwise healthy person under typical conditions should be able to cool down readily and compensate." She adds that it may help to realize that while sweat is a loss to your body, it is one that you can easily replace through hydration to achieve that balance. By understanding what's going on in our bodies, and that's it's normal to sweat during a workout, will help reduce fears.

Fear: Hurting Your Back

Getting injured is a legitimate concern — and that's where proper form comes in. When doing lower body exercises, like squats and lunges, it's important to engage the lower abs to support your back. Pull your naval in towards your spine, and never do exercises that feel like they're pulling on your back. Work out slowly and consciously so that you can notice even the slightest feeling of discomfort in your low back. At the end of your workout, stretch by lying down on your back, and then hugging your knees into your chest for 20 seconds.

Many people believe that exercise can aggravate back pain or make it worse, but working out properly can help strengthen the back and reduce pain. Eric Owens, co-founder of Delos Therapy, who specializes in pain management that involves stretching muscles and fascia with pressure, says, "Strengthening the core with abdominal exercises along with strengthening the back with big compound movements such as the squat are important for a healthy core and healthy body — but remember that strengthening only comes after restoring pliability." He urges people to focus on flexibility and increasing the mobility of the muscles before using strength training to strengthen your back. If you have a back injury, consult your doctor or physical therapist before starting any exercise regimen.

Fear: Pulling a Muscle

Warming up before you work out is just as important as stretching after you work out — and it can help you prevent a pulled muscle. Owens explains what a pulled muscle may feel like: "Typically, it presents as a sharp pain at the location of the strain or tear with subsequent limited range of motion and weakness."

To help prevent this, make sure you stretch properly. For pre-workout stretches, make sure you keep moving and are doing dynamic, active stretches. Try this:

Step forward into a lunge position with your right foot forward. Bend the right knee to stretch the left hip flexor, and then straighten the right leg to stretch the right hamstring. Keep moving back and forth without holding the stretch. Switch sides.

Swing your arms around to stretch your torso. The key is to keep moving during these pre-workout stretches.

Post-workout you can perform static stretches, where you hold them for 20-30 seconds, because your muscles are already warmed up from the workout. Here's an example:

* Move into the same lunge position, but hold it for 20-30 seconds.

* Stretch the hamstring for 20-30 seconds, and switch sides.

Fear: Breaking a Machine

I've had more than one client ask me if I think it's possible to break a machine while working out. Generally they're afraid of stepping onto an elliptical or sitting on a spin bike and breaking it. Of course there is always a small chance that if a piece of equipment is used incorrectly with a lot of force, it can break, but this is highly unlikely. Put this fear aside, and when in doubt, ask an instructor or a personal trainer to help you adjust the bike or elliptical correctly before hopping on.

Fear: Not Accomplishing Your Goals

Do you have that nagging fear that this time recommitting to the gym (and vowing to lose weight) is going to be like all the other times — a one hit wonder? If you're worried about letting yourself down (again), try to break down your goal into smaller incremental steps, like focusing on one workout at a time. Focus on your successes in that single session: Did you push yourself 30 seconds more in cardio, or did you do more reps with your arm exercises? Did you feel less out of breath or stronger during your workout? Track these individual successes, be proud of yourself and bask in the glory of successfully completing it. Then, move on to the next day. Over time, you'll encourage yourself to push harder through each individual exercise session, which will add up to major results in the long term.

Fear: Not Knowing What to Do

If you're worried about looking awkward when you're in between exercises, use the downtime to add in a few small stretches. Try these stretches:

Stand up next to a wall or another machine nearby and stretch your calves. Put your right toes up on the wall or machine, and standing upright lean into the machine or wall to feel a stretch in your right calf. Then switch sides.

Stand up and cross your right ankle over your left knee, and bend the left knee slightly to feel a stretch in the right glute. You can hold onto a machine or the wall for stability.

While you're stretching, you can assess the gym layout, eye different machines or weights that you'd like to use, and mentally make a plan without anyone knowing that you need the extra time to prepare.

Fear: Post-workout pain (that doesn't go away)

If you've suffered from an injury from the gym, you may

be worried about this happening again. To reduce the chances of an injury, ease back into fitness, especially if it's been awhile since you've had a consistent routine. We tend to feel a burst of motivation in the new year, which is great, but jumping into an exercise routine full throttle can lead to injuries that may put you out of commission (and halt your progress altogether), so it's better to start small and gradually increase your intensity.

The good news is that "muscular discomfort or a strain will usually go away in a day or two. Symptoms can include soreness that is localized, bruising, stiffness and weakness," according to New York City-based physical therapist Marianne Ryant. If this symptoms feel familiar, take it easy until the pain subsides. If you've been to group classes, do half of the repetition and half of the lessons suggested? Stand in the back and go at your own pace. If you're doing strength training, cut your weight in half. Same thing with your cardio: cut your speed in half. And beware of symptoms that linger, and of any immediate pain that you felt that was accompanied by a sound (like a snap or pop). These are signs that you should consult a physician.

Think of losing fat, not losing weight

Weight reduction is one of all time's hottest topics. Nowadays everybody seems trying to lose weight. Most diet plans include weight loss, and also use body weight as a measure of fitness success. Even this approach is imprecise.

Your ultimate goal should always be to lose fat, and reducing excess body fat is what you should be concerned about. Weight loss and Fat loss is NOT the same thing! Many people confuse the two terms, often believing that they mean the same, when, in fact, weight loss and fat loss are very different from one another. This write-up will help you understand how weight loss is different than fat loss and how fat loss is far superior to weight loss in almost all ways.

What Is Weight Loss?
(Weight Loss = Muscle Loss + Fat Loss + Water Loss)

Weight loss is attempting to lower your total body weight. It simply refers to a lower number on a scale. Your body weight is composed of all the parts of your body, such as muscles, fat, bones, water, organs, tissues, blood, water, etc. When you lose weight, you lose a little bit of… fat, muscle, and water.

You lose fat but very little, and you lose muscle and some amount of water along with the fat. The higher you reduce your calorie intake, the faster you drop weight, and the more muscle mass you lose.

Do you know your muscle matters? Loss of muscle affects your health and your overall appearance.

When you lose weight too quickly, your body cannot maintain its muscle. Because muscle requires more calories to sustain itself, your body begins to metabolize it to reserve the incoming calories for its survival. It protects its fat stores as a defense mechanism to ensure your survival in case of future famine. Instead, it uses lean tissue or muscle to provide it with calories it needs to keep its vital organs such as your brain, heart, kidneys, and liver functioning. If you reach a point where you have very little fat or muscle, your body will metabolize your organs to keep your brain functioning leading to heart attack, stroke, and liver and kidney failure.

If the body lacks more muscle tissue, the average metabolic rate of the body shrinks. The metabolic rate is the rate the body burns calories at and is determined in part by the amount of muscle.

So the more muscle you have, the higher your metabolic rate; the less muscle you have, the lower your metabolic rate, and the fewer calories you burn. This explains why it is crucial to protect your metabolic rate and not have muscle loss.

Loss of muscle also leads to loss of tone underneath the skin, leaving you soft and unshapely with no form or contour. If you lose weight too rapidly, your skin won't have time to adjust either. Also, muscle is what gives you strength, and loss of it means a weak body. With weight loss, you shrink in size and become a smaller version of yourself with a fragile frame with saggy skin.

Weight loss works in the short run to make you smaller but is temporary, almost everyone rebounds and regains the weight. This forces you to find another diet. And then another one, and another one - because eventually, they'll all fail.

What Is the Loss of Fat?
(Weight Loss = Accumulated Body Fat Loss)

Fat loss attempts to reduce your total body fat-that is the percentage of your total body weight that's made up of fat. The right approach to fat loss is to exercise intelligently and eat smartly in a way that maintains muscle and is focused exclusively on fat loss.

You don't have the strength for now. If you don't feed it and use it, then you lose it. A proper plan with the right combination of cardiovascular resistance training with adequate progression and the right nutrition plan to support it can help you achieve this. Exercise only boosts the process of burning but does not merely melt away the fat on its own if you do not create a deficit and feed the body too much, and it will not touch the stored fuel reserves. On the other hand, if you cut your calories drastically and do not properly feed your muscle or do not exercise and use your muscle, you will lose it. Fat loss is about striking the right balance.

With fat loss, you keep the muscle running high and keep the metabolic rate high. You develop stronger connective tissue as well as tighter skin and stronger bones and joints. You'll be transforming your body with fat loss.

Fat loss is a lifestyle strategy where you give the body what it wants with the pressure of hunger, without depriving and startling it. You get to see steady progress slow but permanent.

It may sound weird, but you may get smaller without having a weight change. It is because you lose body fat as you add muscle. Even when you lose inches, your weight stays the same.

Let's see how it works out.

Fat tissue is not thick and is rather flexible. This takes up lots of room in the body, while the muscle is denser and takes up less space. This space is freed when you lose fat, and you may notice a loss of inch. Gaining in lean muscle mass will even out this lack of fat and weight remains the same while you are doing a regular strength training program. If the muscle takes up less room than fat, you lose inches and start becoming more toned, lean, and shapely.

Consistent strength exercise regimen, then gain in lean muscle mass matches this fat loss and weight stays the same. If the muscle takes up less room than fat, you lose inches and start becoming more toned, lean, and shapely.

Myth: "To suit" means "to lose weight."
Truth: To get fit means to reduce the percentage of your body fat!

CHAPTER 7:THE BENEFITS OF LOS-ING WEIGHT

Losing weight has a range of advantages. It's not easy to lose weight. Some people want a well-shaped body. Others are doing the same for their overall health. Perhaps the long-term utility of weight loss can motivate anyone to take up this activity.

Below are some of the well known weight-loss advantages:
Weight reduction helps prevent hypertension and other heart diseases:

You may call this a three in one benefit of weight loss. Heart diseases and strokes are fatal diseases that account for many American deaths each year. Overweight people are at great risk of having increased deposits of cholesterol and triglycerides in their blood.
Angina is a common heart disease characterized by pain in the chest and a decrease in oxygen pumped to the heart.
Heart diseases and strokes can also cause instant deaths. These usually occur without any warnings and symptoms.
Studies have proven that a small decrease in weight (five to ten percent) can significantly improve your health, and you can save yourself from all these deadly diseases. Besides, this would also help maintain stable blood pressure and regulate the level of cholesterol and triglyceride in your body.

Weight Loss prevents two types of diabetes:

Diabetes is a very serious disease that puts one life in jeopardy. Both type one and type two diabetes are associated with overweight. For diabetes patients, you recommend that you take up regular exercise and weight loss diet to control your blood sugar level. It will also affect the medication that you might be taking currently. You should increase your physical activities. Start walking, jogging, or dancing. This will help both in the circulation of your blood and the reduction of weight.

Weight Loss Reduces the Risk of Cancer:

Obesity is also associated with different kinds of cancer. For women, the common types of cancer linked with being overweight include gallbladder, ovary, breast, uterus, and colon cancer. This is only meant to keep you informed about the hazards that you risk yourself into by not reducing weight. Men may also develop cancer due to obesity. Men are more susceptible to cancers of the colon, rectum, and prostate. It is recommended that you reduce your weight besides avoiding diets rich in fat and cholesterol.

Weight Loss Prevents Sleep Apnea:

Reducing your weight could also help you to prevent sleep apnea or reduce it considerably. Sleep apnea is a disorder in which one stops breathing temporarily. It lasts for a brief period and is followed by heavy snoring. It can cause drowsiness and fatigue during the day. Overweight people are also at risk of heart failure due to sleep apnea. Removing those extra layers of fat could help eliminate this disorder.

Weight Loss Reduces Osteoarthritis Pain:

When a person is overweight, knee joints, lower back, and hips exert a lot to carry around. It is believed that these body parts have to exert up to 2-3 times more than normal. This causes stress and tension in joints. Reducing your weight will provide relief to these joints by decreasing the load they have to carry. This helps reduce osteo-arthritis pain.

Lose fat and gain muscle without cardio. Discover the cardio, free fat loss work

There are some general instructions, thumb rules, and, ways to interpret a diet plan which will help you to determine, once and for all, whether it is the correct diet for you. You do not like what I have to say, and this is another fast remedy under no expectations, "loose 100 lbs. in 20 days," guide of some kind. However, if you're sick and tired of being lost, tired of getting the weight off just to bring it back on, and tired of asking how to take the first steps to determine the correct diet for you which will result in lasting weight loss, then this is the write-up that might change your life.

Does "The Test" pass your diet?

And what's the biggest reason diets fail in the long run, most of all? Explanatory number one is drum roll, Long-term lack of commitment. The numbers are not lying; it will be regained by the vast majority of people who lose weight-and often exceed that which they lost. You knew you didn't?

Yet what do you do to prevent it? Here's another reality check: practically any diet you choose that embraces the simple principle of "eating" more calories than you eat-the well-accepted "calories out" slogan-can lead you to lose weight. They all work to some degree: Atkins-style, no carb diets, low-fat high carb diets, all sorts of fad diets-it just does n't matter in the short term.

When you aim to drop a certain weight fast, then pick one and follow it. I'm guaranteeing you'll lose some weight. Studies generally find that after six months to a year, any of the commercial weight-loss diets will get off about the same amount. New research, for example, showed Atkins' diet, the Slim-Fast method, the Weight Watchers Simple Points system, and Rosemary Conley's Eat Yourself Slim diet were all similarly successful.

Other studies comparing other popular diets concluded essentially the same. For instance, a study comparing the Atkins diet, the Ornish diet, Weight Watchers, and The Zone Diet found that they were essentially the same in their ability to take off the weight after a year.
Note what I have said about diets missing number one excuse, which is a lack of compliance. In this recent study, the lead researcher stated:
"Our trial found that adherence level was the primary predictor of weight loss rather than diet type."

Translated, it's not what diet they chose per se, but their ability to adhere to a diet that predicted their success in weight loss. "But will some diets be better than others, right?" Are some diets better than others? Definitely. Truly. A few other diets are healthier than the others, some diets are better for preserving lean body mass, some diets are better for suppressing appetite, and there are many different diets. While most common diets will work to take the weight off, it is abundantly clear that adhering to the diet is the most important aspect to keep the weight off over the long term.

What is a diet?
A diet is a form of weight-loss at short notice. Long-term weight loss is the result of an enhancement in diets. We're talking with lifetime weight control, not fast weight loss repair here. I don't like the term diet, because it's a short-term attempt at weight loss vs. a lifestyle change. Want to fast lose a bunch of weight? Heck, I 'm going to give you the information about how to do it here and now for no charge.

Eat 12 scrambled egg whites, a whole grapefruit, and a gallon of water twice a day for the next 90 to 120 days. You will lose a lot of weight. Will it be Healthy? NO. When you're done with this diet, will the weight stay off? No chance. No possibility. Will the weight you lose be muscle, water, bone, and (hopefully!) some fat? The argument is, there are many diets out there that are completely capable of keeping weight off you, but you have to question yourself before contemplating some food program intended to reduce weight:

"Is this one way I can live long-term?"

What brings me to my test: I call it the test, "Can I eat this way for the rest of my life?" I know, it's not just rolling your tongue off, but it's getting the point across.

The message here is that whatever food diet you choose for weight loss must be part of a lifestyle change that you will be able to follow forever. That is, if it's not a way you can live forever, even after you reach your target weight, it's useless.

Therefore, several fad diets you see out are removed automatically, so you don't have to think about them. The problem is not whether the diet can be successful in the short term, but whether it will be practiced indefinitely as a way to live for a lifetime. A failure formula and the cause of the well-established yo-yo diet phenomenon is to go from eating "their" way back to eating "their" way once you hit your target weight. Bottom line: there are no short cuts, no free lunch, and just a dedication to dietary change can hold the weight off in the long term. I realize that is not what most people want to hear, but it is the truth, like it or not.

Teach Fish to a Man

A well-known Chinese proverb is, teach a man fishing, and you will feed him for life.

That expression suits well with the next important step of determining what diet routine you will adopt to lose weight effectively. Does the diet plan you are considering teach you how to eat in the long term, or does it give you details on spoon feed? Does the diet depend on special bars, beverages, vitamins, or pre-made foods in their stock?

Let's do another study diet A vs. diet B. Diet A will supply you with their meals, as well as their special drinks or bars, to consume and tell you exactly when to consume them. Within two months, you should lose-say-30 lbs. Diet B will attempt to help you understand what foods you should consume, how much calories you need to consume, why you need to eat them, and ultimately seek to help educate you about how to diet as part of a total lifestyle change that will encourage you to make healthier decisions about your nutrition. Diet B causes a sluggish, gradual weight loss of 8-10 lbs every month for the next six months and holds the weight off because you now learn how to eat well.

Recall the Chinese proverb. Both diets will help you get weight loss. Just one diet, though, will teach you how to be self-reliant after your practice is over. Diet A is better, to be sure, which induces greater weight loss than diet B, which diet B takes longer and needs more thought and preparation on your part. When diet A is done, though, you are right back where you started, and you were given no fishing skills. Diet companies don't make their profits by training you to eat, they make their money by tossing you an eat, and you have to focus on them forever or come back to them after you get all the weight back.

Consequently, diet B is superior to allow you to succeed where other diets have failed, with knowledge gained that you can apply for the long term. Diet systems that aim to feed you a diet spoon without having to show you how to eat without their help and/or dependent on their drinks, chips, cookies, or pre-made foods is another diet that you can remove from your preference list.

Diet plans which offer weight loss by having to drink their product for several meals accompanied by a 'functional dinner;' diets that encourage you to eat their specific cookies for most of the meals along with their pre-planned menu; or diets that try to get you to eat their bars, drinks or pre-made meals belong to the aforementioned diet A. They are easy to follow but, long-term, destined for failure. They both miss the "Should I live this way for the rest of my life?" test unless you believe you should eat cookies and shakes for the rest of your life... The bottom line here is, if the dietary strategy you use to lose weight, whether from a novel, a seminar, a clinic, or an e-book, doesn't show you how to diet, it's a failure long-term weight loss and should be stopped.

The missing link to weight loss over the long term

We are now heading for another test to help you select a long-term weight loss nutrition program, and it doesn't involve nutrition. The missing link to weight loss in the long term is exercise. Exercise is a key component of weight loss in the long term. Many diet plans have no element of exercise, meaning they're losers for long-term weight loss from the very beginning. Any program focusing on weight loss but not including a comprehensive exercise plan is like buying a tireless car or a wingless plane. People who have succeeded in keeping the weight off have incorporated exercise predominantly into their lives, and the studies that look at people who have successfully lost weight and kept it off invariably find these people consistent with their diet and exercise plans.

I won't list all the benefits of regular exercise here, but regular exercise has positive effects on your weight, helps you to eat more calories while still in a calorie deficit, and can help preserve lean body mass (LBM) that is essential to your health and metabolism.

SideBar: Short comment on workout:

Any exercise is better than no preparation. However, not all exercises are done together, such as diet programs, and many people still use the wrong kind of exercise to improve their weight loss efforts. They will, for example, do aerobics exclusively and ignore the resistance training. Resistance exercise is an integral aspect of weight loss as it produces balanced metabolic muscle, increases the development of 24-hour energy, and delivers health benefits beyond aerobics.

However, the reader will remember that I said fat loss and not weight loss. While in this piece, I use the word 'weight loss,' mostly because most people recognize it's a common term. However, a well-designed diet and exercise plan's true emphasis, and the target will be on fat loss, not weight loss. The wrong approach is to focus on weight loss, which can include a loss of essential muscle, water, and even bone. Losing weight and maintaining the all-important lean body mass is the goal. Bottom line: the type of exercise, the speed of the exercise, the length of the exercise, etc., are important factors when attempting to lose FAT while maintaining the exercise.

The psychological dimension of why individuals with long-term weight loss struggle to be successful is not discussed by many diet programs out there. Nonetheless, there are also a few reports that looked into exactly that. The psychological factor for a long-term weight loss is the most significant in many ways, and the most understated part is certainly.

Researchers compared the psychological features of people who have successfully held the weight off to those who have lost the weight find significant distinctions in these two categories. A case that looked at 28 obese women who had lost weight but regained the weight they had lost, compared to 28 women who had lost weight and maintained their weight for at least one year, and 20 women with steady weight in the healthier range found the women who regained weight:

- Had a propensity to measure self-worth concerning weight and shape
- Were lacking vigilance on weight control
- Had a dichotomous (black and white) style of thinking
- Had a tendency to regulate mood using eating.

Researchers concluded:
"The results suggest that some explanation for psychological factors may be given as to why many people with obesity are regaining weight after a successful weight loss."
This particular study was conducted on women, so it illustrates some of the different psychological issues that women have-but do not make any mistakes here-men have their psychological problems that may hinder their long-term attempts to lose weight.
Recent male and female research found personality characteristics such as "setting ambitious weight targets, weak coping strategies or problem-solving abilities, and low self-efficacy" also indicate long-term disappointment with weight loss.
On the other hand, psychological characteristics common to people who have experienced positive long-term weight loss include. ".. an internal motivation to lose weight, social support, improved coping strategies and ability to cope with life stress, self-efficacy, flexibility, assuming responsibility in life, and more psychological strength and stability overall."
The key point of this segment is that psychology plays a major role in determining whether people are successful with weight loss over the long term. If it is not addressed

as part of the overall plan, it can be the factor that makes or breaks your success.

However, this isn't an area that most nutrition programs can and should not be expected to address adequately. In general, better programs try to help with motivation, setting goals, and support.

If you are among the groups, who have failed to maintain their weight in the above charts, in the long run, realize that you will try to address these issues through therapy, neighborhood activities, etc. Do not expect any weight loss plan to address this issue sufficiently but look for services that aim to offer encouragement, target setting, and tools to keep you on track.

So why don't you see this sort of truthful knowledge more often about the effects of weight loss in the long term? Let's be honest here, and it's not the easiest way to say the truth to sell drinks, shakes, magazines, vitamins, and services. Hell, if everybody who read this book followed it by some miracle, and sent it on to millions of other people who followed it, makers of such products could quickly be in financial trouble.

So let's recall what's been learned here: the big picture realities of permanent weight loss and how you can look at a weight loss program and decide for yourself whether it is based on what's covered below:

- Successful weight loss is not about seeking a fast diet but about sticking to improvements in the lifestyle that include eating and exercise
- Any program for weight loss you choose must pass the test "Can I eat that way for the rest of my life?"
- Ideally, the weight management plan you chose will

teach you how to diet and be self-reliant, so you can make better long-term food decisions.

- For your long-term results, the weight loss plan you chose will not leave you relying on commercial chips, drinks, vitamins, or pre-made foods.

- The weight loss plan you select needs to have an appropriate workout portion.

- The weight loss program you choose should help with motivation, goal setting, and support

I want to take this last section to add a few more points and clarity. The advice given above is not for everyone, for example. This is not meant for those who have dialed in their diet, including professional bodybuilders and other athletes who benefit from relatively dramatic dietary changes such as 'off-season' and 'pre-contest' etc.

The piece is also not meant for those with medical problems that may be on a particular diet to treat or manage a specific medical condition. The book is meant for the average person who wants to get off the merry-go-round diet of Yo-Yo once and for all. It will cover millions of people as that is probably 99 percent of the population.

 That doesn't mean you're going to diet for the rest of your life and have nothing to look forward to but hunger. What it does mean, though, is that you'll continue to remember to eat better well after you hit your target weight, and that way of eating shouldn't be a massive change from how you lived to lose weight first. Once you reach your target weight-and/or body fat levels, you're going to go into a maintenance phase that usually has more calories and food choices, including occasional treatments like pizza or anything.

Maintenance diets are a rational continuation of the diet that you used to lose weight, but they're not based on the regimen that you adopted that takes the weight first!

CHAPTER 8:   KETO DIET AND WEIGHT LOSS

If you've had an urge to lose those extra pounds, you may have tried a ketogenic diet known as the Keto diet. It is a popular weight-loss plan promising substantial weight loss in a short time.

But the diet is not a magic tool for weight loss, far from most people believe it to be. It takes time, like any other diet, to see results, and requires a lot of adjustment and tracking.

Keto diet is aimed at putting your body in ketosis. In general, this diet plan is low in carb with a high intake of healthy fats, vegetables, and enough protein. There's also an emphasis on this diet on eliminating highly processed foods and sugars.

There are several types of diets with Keto: standard diets with ketogenic, cyclical, targeted, and high protein. The disparity therein depends on the consumption of carb. The standard ketogenic diet is low in carb, high in fat, and most recommended is adequate protein.

Is the Keto Diet healthy?

Some Keto diet critics say it isn't healthy because of the emphasis on high-fat content consumption. That's motivated by the myth that fats are bad for you. Quite the opposite, healthy fats are actually quite good for you.

You get lots of fats from healthy sources such as avocado, nuts, fish, butter, eggs, coconut oil, palm oil, chia seeds, and red meat.

How does the Keto diet help with weight loss?

So how does the keto diet work and help you lose excess pounds in your body? The body uses energy from carbs and sugars for feeding body movements while on a high carb diet. When you take a ketogenic diet, minimal amounts of carbs and sugar are supplied to the body.

With a reduced supply of sugar and carbs, the glucose levels in the body are depleted, causing the body to look for alternative energy sources. Consequently, the body becomes stored fats for energy, which is why the diet of Keto leads to weight loss.

This disorder is called ketosis since the body uses fats for energy other than carbohydrates. When your body enters ketosis, ketones were produced as the source of fuel, rather than depending on glucose. Ketones and glucose are the only two sources of energy that fuel the brain.

Advantages of Ketosis and Keto diet:

Besides just helping in weight loss, it also comes with other health benefits to put the body in ketosis. Here are a few of them:

- Enhanced mental clarity
- Improved physical energy
- Steady blood sugar levels which make it a good remedy for epilepsy and diabetes
- Improved and enhanced skin tones
- Lower cholesterol levels
- Hormone regulation especially in women

The Ketogenic diet is among the easiest weight loss diets you can try to improve general health. The diet can also be used for children who are overweight. Numerous studies support the diet showing significant results, especially when coupled with exercise.

Tips and Exercise Plans to Lose Weight

There are several options to easily lose weight and immediately melt the fat away. Most of them, however, leave you unsatisfied as one realizes that shortcuts to weight loss are not long term sustainable. Loss of weight is a combination of a well-formulated diet plan and a rigorous exercise regime. When you're curious how to reduce weight here are a few easy tips for weight management and weight loss and weight control workout programs-

1. Work your spirit out.

Weight loss refers to a good diet, a rigorous exercise regime, but, most importantly, to mental conviction. Once you embark on a weight loss journey, take a mental note of why you are taking this step and have a justification for keeping you going to avoid binge eating from catering to those cravings.

2. Avoid food that is high in sugar.

Insulin is the fat storage compound in our bodies, and insulin is activated from sugary foods such as sweets. This instantly increases our blood sugar levels, which in turn contributes to fat storage. Lowering insulin also acts as a detox to the body enabling the kidneys to expel any excess sodium or nitrates that may cause bloating. Cutting out fizzy drinks completely is important.

3. Don't just take a food group out.

The weight loss industry turns one or the other food group the worst for the body every year. As part of our diet, it is possible to have all the fats, sugars, and proteins. Protein-rich foods have been shown to boost your metabolism and also reduce cravings

4. Water is salvation to you.

Stay hydrated with water and other fluids all day long. To prevent all that bloating, one must drink at least eight glasses of water a day. Just after you wake up, it is recommended to have a glass of water with lemon in it.

5. Fiber is essential to a healthy gut.

Food like vegetables is high in fiber, preventing constipation and promptly helping one get a flat belly. This also assists in the long-term strengthening of the digestive system and improved digestion.

6. Stay out of fad diets.

Today's market is flooded with diets like the GM diet, Atkins diet, and Keto diet, all of which have very serious long-term consequences for our bodies. Anything that comes quickly goes fast, so remember to be patient and eat all but in moderation.

Diet Weight Loss plan:

Below is a regular diet that you can use for weight loss.

Breakfast: 3 egg whites OR fruit and cup of green tea with oatmeal.

Mid-morning snack: 150 gm of chicken fried in vinegar and soy OR 1 6-inch fresh or grilled corn tortilla (onions, green bell peppers, and tomatoes) and non-added salsa.

Lunch: Grilled Roasted Fish OR 2 Cups Wrapped in Balsamic Vinegar Blended Greens with 1 Cup of Other Vegetables

Midsummer afternoon snack: a chickpea salad Plus a banana and one apple

Dinner: Any protein (Tofu, chicken, fish, etc.) OR fresh ingredient salad

Workout plan to lose weight:

Need some exercise to lose weight? Follow an exercise plan that lets you try out a new thing every day. Engage like playing in fast cardio, Zumba, jumping, but even visit the gym to drop weight. Holding the muscle mass is essential, and it burns fat even after the exercise is done. A perfect way to burn a solid 1000 calories is a fast exercise of high-intensity strength training.

If you obey the above points, you're bound to healthily

lose weight! A diet and some exercise do the trick.